Magnet Therapy

Magnetic therapy for Different Ailments, How it Works, History, Indications, and Contraindications

Dani Twain

Copyright Notice

All rights reserved. No part of this publication may be reproduced, stored in a retrieval system or transmitted in any form or by any means, including electronic, digital, mechanical, photocopying, audio recording, printing or otherwise, without written permission from the publisher or the author.

Contents

Chapter 1

What is Magnetic Therapy?

Magnetic therapy, also known as magnetotherapy, is a type of treatment that uses magnets to help heal the body. There are different kinds of magnetic fields used in this therapy, such as constant, variable, pulsating, rotating, and pulsed magnetic fields. The pulsed magnetic fields are considered the most effective for treating people because our body tissues respond best to them.

This therapy works by using electromagnetic fields to encourage the body to produce and use bioactive molecules more effectively.

Why is Magnetic Therapy Useful?
Magnetic therapy offers several health benefits:

- **Improves Brain Circulation:** Helps blood flow better in the brain.
- **Reduces Muscle Tension:** Relaxes the walls of veins and arteries, lowering tension.
- **Aids Stroke Recovery:** Speeds up the process of regaining limb movement after a stroke.
- **Enhances Healing:** Boosts the repair processes in muscles and nerve tissues.

- **Reduces Pain:** Lessens pain in the back and joints.

- **Improves Blood Circulation:** Enhances blood flow and tissue blood supply.

- **Improves Blood Quality:** Enhances the structure and viscosity of the blood.

- **Boosts Immunity:** Strengthens the immune system, stimulates collagen production, and improves tissue nutrition.

Chapter 2

The Basics of Magnetic Fields

Magnetic fields are everywhere, but many people don't think much about them. By learning the basics of magnetic fields, you can better understand their properties and uses in daily life.

In this chapter, we'll explore what magnetic fields are, their characteristics, and how they impact our everyday activities. Get ready to discover the fascinating world of magnetic fields!

What is a Magnetic Field?

A magnetic field is an area in space where magnetic forces can be detected. These forces are generated by the movement of electric charges, such as those in the atoms that make up everything around us.

One key feature of a magnetic field is its polarity. Just like a magnet has a north and south pole, a magnetic field also has opposite poles that either attract or repel each other based on their orientation.

Magnetic fields are not just scientific curiosities; they have many practical uses in our daily lives.

Magnetic fields are also found in nature. They play a crucial role in the migration of birds and the formation of the aurora borealis (northern lights). Even the Earth has a magnetic field, which protects us from harmful solar radiation and helps guide the migration patterns of many animals.

The Science Behind Magnetic Fields

A magnetic field consists of invisible lines of force around a magnet. These lines result from the alignment of particles within the material, creating a net magnetic field.

External factors can also influence a magnetic field. For instance, a moving electric charge creates a magnetic field around it. Similarly, when an electric current passes through a wire, it generates a circular magnetic field around the wire. These interactions help us understand magnetism better.

Even though scientists don't fully understand all the complexities of magnetic fields, their importance in modern technology is undeniable. You can't see magnetic fields with your eyes, but they play a vital role in shaping our universe.

What Are Magnetic Field Lines?

Magnetic field lines are a visual representation of the magnetic field around a magnet or a current-carrying wire. These lines help us understand the strength and direction of the magnetic field and how it interacts with other magnets or conductive materials.

The magnetic field lines of a magnet always extend from the north pole to the south pole, forming a continuous loop. The density of these lines indicates the strength of the magnetic field: closely spaced lines represent a strong field, while widely spaced lines indicate a weak field.

Understanding magnetic fields and their properties can deepen your appreciation for this invisible but powerful force that influences many aspects of our world.

Properties of Magnetic Fields

Magnetic fields are invisible forces that play a crucial role in many scientific mysteries. Let's explore their properties and how they work.

Direction and Strength

Magnetic fields have both direction and strength. They are often represented as lines of force that flow from the north pole to the south pole of a magnet. The field's strength decreases as you move farther away from the magnet.

Polarity

Polarity is another key property of magnetic fields. Like poles (north-north or south-south) repel each other, while opposite poles (north-south) attract. This is why magnets can either attract or repel each other based on their orientation.

The magnetic field created by a wire carrying an electric current can be clockwise or counterclockwise, depending on the direction of the current flow.

Induction

Magnetic fields can induce electrical currents in conductors, a phenomenon known as electromagnetic induction. This is how generators produce electricity. Similarly, electric currents can produce magnetic fields, which is the principle behind how motors work.

How to Measure Magnetic Fields

There are several ways to measure the strength and direction of a magnetic field:

- Magnetometer: This instrument detects changes in magnetic fields using coils and sensors. It can measure everything from Earth's natural magnetic field to man-made electromagnetic fields.

- Hall Effect Sensor: This device measures electrical current flowing through a conductor in the presence of a magnetic field.

- Fluxgate Magnetometer: This technique uses an alternating current passed through ferromagnetic-wrapped coils to measure magnetic fields.

Magnetic Fields vs. Electromagnetic Fields

While magnetic and electromagnetic fields share some similarities, they have key differences:

- Magnetic Fields: Created by moving electric charges and measured in teslas or gauss.
- Electromagnetic Fields: A combination of electric and magnetic fields, measured in hertz or decibels.

Electromagnetic fields can exist without magnetic fields, but magnetic fields cannot exist without electric currents. Magnetic fields are generated by the motion of charged particles, while electromagnetic fields result from the interaction of electric and magnetic fields.

What is Magnetic Field Mapping?

Magnetic field mapping is a technique used to visualize and measure the strength and direction of magnetic fields in a specific area. A magnetometer, which detects and measures magnetic fields, is commonly used for this purpose. Magnetic field mapping is used in various fields, including geology, physics, and engineering.

- **Geology:** To map Earth's magnetic field and study tectonic plate movements.

- **Physics:** To understand material properties.

- **Engineering:** To design electronic devices and identify magnetic field issues in equipment.

Purpose of a Magnetic Field

Magnetic fields have many important uses in our world, from navigation to powering electronics.

- Navigation: Earth's magnetic field helps animals like birds and bees navigate long distances. It is also the basis for compasses used in navigation. Magnetic fields assist in aviation and marine navigation, helping pilots and sailors stay on course.

- Electricity Generation and Transmission: Generators and transformers use magnetic fields to produce and transfer electrical energy.

- Medical Applications: MRI machines use powerful magnetic fields to create images of the body's internal structures, aiding in the diagnosis and treatment of various medical conditions.

Magnetic fields are an essential part of modern life, helping us understand and interact with the world around us.

How Can You Define Magnetism?

Magnetism is a natural force that makes certain materials attract or repel each other. When an object is magnetic, it creates a magnetic field around itself, which can affect other magnetic objects nearby. Learning about magnetism helps us understand many everyday phenomena and its many applications in technology and industry.

Magnetism is involved in various aspects of daily life, such as the attraction of a compass needle to the Earth's magnetic field. It is also essential in industries like electronics, transportation, and energy production. Common uses of magnetism include electric motors, generators, MRI machines, and compasses. Additionally, magnetism is used to separate different types of metals and store data on computer hard drives.

What Are the Characteristics of Magnetic Force?

Magnetic force is the force that magnets or magnetic fields exert on other magnets or magnetic materials. Here are the main characteristics of magnetic force:

Attraction and Repulsion

- Attraction: Opposite poles (north and south) of magnets attract each other.
- Repulsion: Like poles (north-north or south-south) repel each other.

Direction

- The direction of the magnetic force is always perpendicular to the motion of the magnetic field.

Strength

- The strength of the magnetic force is proportional to the strength of the magnetic field and the amount of magnetic material.

Distance

- Magnetic force decreases as the distance between the magnets increases.

Inverse Square Law

- The strength of the magnetic force follows the inverse square law. If the distance between two magnets doubles, the force between them decreases by a factor of four.

Conclusion

From the Earth's magnetic field to the fields created by everyday magnets, magnetic fields are a crucial part of our lives. By learning about magnetic fields and their unique properties, we can gain a deeper understanding of this fascinating natural phenomenon and its importance in technology and industry.

Chapter 3

History of Magnetic Therapy

Ancient Beginnings

The use of magnetized stones for healing dates back to around 4000 BC. By 2000 BC, Chinese doctors were using magnets to treat acupuncture points. In Ancient Greece, Hippocrates, the "Father of Medicine," reportedly used magnets to treat headaches and other pains. Although detailed records from ancient times are scarce, it is clear that people recognized the healing power of magnets long ago.

From the Middle Ages to the 20th Century

Magnetotherapy saw significant developments starting in the 16th century. The Swiss physician Paracelsus used magnets to treat mental disorders and seizures. This practice was continued by the German doctor Franz Mesmer in the 18th century, although knowledge about magnetic fields and magnetism was still limited.

Interest in magnetic fields grew in the 19th century. The English scientist Michael Faraday made major contributions by discovering electromagnetic induction, diamagnetism, and electrolysis. He was the first to prove that a changing magnetic field creates an electric field.

In the early 20th century, Russian engineer Georges Lakhovsky created the "radio-cellular oscillator," a device producing a range of therapeutic frequencies. He believed each cell oscillated at a specific frequency and proposed using his device to treat cancer, though this idea was not scientifically validated.

From the 20th Century to the Present Day

Modern magnetotherapy began to take shape around the turn of the 19th and 20th centuries. Nikola Tesla's discoveries about the relationship between electricity and magnetic fields, including the rotating magnetic field, laid the groundwork for many inventions. He also invented the standard magnetic loop coil, used in all

PEMF (Pulsed Electromagnetic Field) systems.

The first PEMF devices emerged in the Czech Republic in the 1980s, where complex methods of static magnetic therapy were developed. PEMF therapy soon spread to other European countries and continued to be refined. In the same decade, the first FDA-approved PEMF system for treating nonunion fractures was introduced. By the late 1990s, PEMF therapy was widely used.

Today, magnetic therapy continues to evolve with advancements in technology. It is used to treat various conditions, including those affecting the musculoskeletal system. The continuous improvement of devices and methods ensures that magnetic therapy remains a valuable tool in modern medicine.

Chapter 4

How Does Magnetic Therapy Work?

A common question among those new to Magnetic Therapy is, "How does Magnetic Therapy work?" Experts have different theories and beliefs about how this natural therapy functions. Although we've learned a lot about magnets and their use in alternative therapy, there's still much to discover. Scientists and researchers are working hard to answer this question.

We know that magnets emit a static magnetic field similar to the Earth's magnetic field, which is essential for life and health. The energy field created by biomagnets (healing magnets) helps the body balance and heal itself.

How Magnets Work

In 1954, Linus Pauling won the Nobel Prize in Chemistry for discovering the magnetic properties of hemoglobin, the part of red blood cells that contains iron.

The most common theory is that the magnetic field attracts the iron in hemoglobin, increasing blood flow and circulation. This increase in circulation boosts the amount of oxygen available to the body, strengthens the immune system, and reduces toxins. As a result, pain and inflammation are lessened, and the body's natural healing process is sped up.

Ancient people observed this magnetic phenomenon and benefited from it for over four thousand years without fully understanding how it worked. Perhaps we can follow their example and focus on the benefits of this holistic therapy.

The Normal Healing Process

Healing typically follows a sequence:

1. Immediate Response: Blood platelets stop the bleeding by promoting blood vessel constriction, releasing clotting factors, and forming clots from fibrin. They also attract inflammatory cells to the wound.

2. Inflammatory Reaction: This occurs within 2 to 3 days. Leukocytes, including macrophages, arrive and release enzymes and mediators. They clean the wound by removing bacterial residues, dead cells, and fragments.

3. Fibroblast Activity: Fibroblasts produce collagen and other components of the extracellular matrix to fill the wound. New blood vessels form, and keratinocytes from the wound edges migrate to cover the wound. A new scar should be protected from the sun to prevent permanent pigmentation.

Magnetic Therapy and Collagen

Magnetic therapy, known for pain relief, also aids in healing. The static magnetic field of a magnet stimulates the secretion of type I collagen in the dermis. To use magnets for healing, place them near the wound with opposite poles (north and south) on either side. Increase the number of magnet pairs if needed.

Magnetic Therapy Backed by Research

Research has shown that magnetic therapy benefits both chronic and acute conditions. Modern science is still exploring how and why magnets work, but like electricity or driving a car, you don't need to understand it fully to benefit from it.

Researchers have found that permanent magnets can speed up the body's natural healing process, accelerating post-surgery recovery and wound healing. Clinicians and researchers report an impressive 80 to 90 percent success rate in pain reduction. Biomagnetic research has also shown that permanent magnets can restore energy, boost the immune system, and improve sleep.

Holistic Benefits

Magnetic therapy provides physical, mental, emotional, and spiritual benefits beyond pain relief. It can help with a variety of health problems, including diabetes, depression, insomnia, and chronic fatigue syndrome (CFS). Due to its balancing effect on the body, magnetic therapy can assist in achieving holistic health.

Chapter 5

Health Conditions with Magnetic Therapy

Magnetic Therapy for ENT Diseases

Magnetic therapy is used to treat various diseases, including those affecting the ear, nose, and throat (ENT). Here's how it works and its benefits:

How Magnetic Therapy Works

1. Magnetizing Water Molecules:

   - The human body is about 60-70% water. When exposed to a magnetic field, the water molecules in tissues, blood, and lymph become "magnetized."

- This activation boosts cellular metabolism, normalizes redox processes, and increases enzyme activity.

2. Improving Circulation and Metabolism:

- This therapy enhances blood flow and metabolic processes both in the targeted area and throughout the body.

Effects of Magnetic Therapy

- Reduces Swelling and Pain: Helps alleviate discomfort and inflammation.

- Stimulates Tissue Regeneration: Promotes healing of body tissues.

- Decreases Blood Viscosity: Has a hypocoagulating effect.

- Boosts Immune System: Increases overall body tone and immune activity.

- Calms the Nervous System: Provides a sedative effect.

- Enhances Other Treatments: When combined with medication, acupuncture, manual therapy, and massage, it enhances their effectiveness, shortens treatment time, and extends periods of remission.

Advantages of Magnetic Therapy

- Penetrates Non-Metallic Materials: The magnetic field can pass through clothing, bandages, cotton, wool, and plaster without losing its benefits.

- Minimal Sensations: Patients usually don't feel anything during the procedure, though some might feel warmth or a tingling sensation.

- Safe for All Ages: Well tolerated by elderly patients and those with poor health.

- Easy to Use: No special training or complex equipment needed, saving time and making it cost-effective compared to other physiotherapy methods.

Types of Magnetic Therapy and Their Benefits

1. Low-Frequency Magnetic Therapy:

   - Vasoactive: Normalizes the tone and diameter of blood vessels.

   - Trophic: Improves metabolic processes.

   - Anti-inflammatory: Reduces inflammation, pain, and spasms.

   - Healing: Stimulates reparative processes.

   - Best for chronic pain conditions.

2. High-Intensity Pulsed Magnetic Therapy:

   - Reduces Swelling and Pain: Provides significant relief.

- Myostimulation: Restores muscle tone and nerve conduction.

- Ideal for acute pain (like injuries, wounds, or post-surgery) and motor or sensory disorders.

Indications for Magnetic Therapy

Magnetic therapy is used for:

- Musculoskeletal Disorders: Osteochondrosis, intervertebral hernias, arthritis, fractures.

- Nervous System Issues: Stroke aftermath, neuritis, neuralgia, migraines.

- Respiratory Diseases: Bronchitis, asthma, pneumonia.

- Cardiovascular Problems: Hypertension, atherosclerosis, varicose veins.

- Digestive Disorders: Ulcers, gastritis, colitis.

- Excretory System Ailments: Cystitis, prostatitis, pyelonephritis.

- Gynecological Diseases

- Endocrine Disorders: Diabetes, gout.

- Eye Diseases

- Allergies: Including skin-related allergies.

- ENT Diseases: Sinusitis, rhinitis, otitis media.

Magnetic therapy offers a non-invasive, safe, and effective way to treat various conditions, providing numerous health benefits.

Magnetic Therapy for Ear, Nose, and Throat (ENT) Diseases

ENT diseases are some of the most common reasons people visit doctors. There are hundreds of different ENT conditions, often caused by bacterial and viral infections. These diseases can also be symptoms of other health problems.

Treating ENT Diseases

Treatment for ENT diseases usually includes:

- Medications: Antibiotics, antivirals, and drugs to relieve symptoms.

- Physical Therapy: Techniques to reduce symptoms like swelling, pain, and inflammation.

Physical Therapy Methods

Physical therapy for ENT diseases includes various techniques:

- Heat Therapy: Reduces inflammation and pain.

- Magnetic Fields: Uses magnetic energy to help heal and reduce symptoms.

- Light Therapy: Uses light to treat various conditions.

- Electrotherapy: Uses electrical energy to stimulate healing.

Benefits of Magnetic Therapy

Research has shown that magnetic therapy is effective in treating ENT diseases. It has anti-inflammatory, decongestant, pain-relieving, and allergy-reducing effects. Magnetic therapy works by:

- Improving Blood Flow: Enhances circulation and reduces swelling.

- Reducing Inflammation: Helps to decrease inflammation and pain.

- Stabilizing Cell Membranes: Reduces allergic reactions and stabilizes cells.

- Enhancing Microcirculation: Increases capillary blood flow, which helps in healing.

How Magnetic Therapy Works

- **Magnetic Fields and Blood Flow:** Low-frequency magnetic fields (up to 30 mT) improve blood flow and circulation, reducing swelling and enhancing healing.

- Anti-Allergic Effects: Magnetic therapy helps control allergic reactions and stabilize cell membranes, making it effective for conditions like allergic rhinitis.

Contraindications

Magnetic therapy should not be used in certain conditions, including:

- Bleeding Disorders: Conditions that increase bleeding risk.

- Cancer: Active cancer or benign tumors in the affected area.

- Low Blood Pressure: Severe hypotension.

- Recent Heart Attack or Stroke: Early recovery period.

- High Blood Pressure: Uncontrolled hypertension (above 150 mmHg).

- Implanted Devices: Pacemakers or metal implants (except dental).

- Fever: Body temperature over 38°C.

- Infections: Active infections.

- Pregnancy and Menstruation: During treatment.

- Epilepsy and Mental Illnesses: These conditions.

Treatment Procedure

Before starting magnetic therapy, you need to consult with a physiotherapist to ensure it's safe for you. The treatment procedure is straightforward:

1. Preparation: No special preparation needed.

2. Positioning: You sit in a chair or lie on a couch.

3. Application: Inductors or solenoids are placed on the affected area.

4. Duration: Each session lasts 15-30 minutes.

5. Frequency: Sessions are held daily or every other day for 10-15 treatments.

Follow-Up

You may need to see the physiotherapist again to evaluate the effectiveness of the treatment and make any necessary adjustments.

Magnetic therapy offers a non-invasive and effective way to treat ENT diseases, helping to reduce symptoms and promote healing.

Magnetotherapy in Pediatric Physiotherapy – Effectiveness and Reliability

Magnetic therapy is a popular treatment in pediatric physiotherapy. It uses either alternating or pulsating low-frequency magnetic fields with electromagnets or a constant magnetic field with permanent magnets.

Benefits of Magnetic Therapy

Magnetic therapy has several medicinal effects:

- Anti-inflammatory: Reduces inflammation.
- Lymphatic Drainage: Helps reduce swelling.
- Vasodilator: Widens blood vessels.
- Trophic-Stimulating: Enhances growth and repair of tissues.

- Hypotensive: Lowers blood pressure.

Therapeutic effects include improved blood circulation and metabolism, reduced swelling, and pain relief. Magnetic fields can penetrate through fabrics like cotton and wool, as well as plaster, without losing effectiveness. This means treatments can be done through thin clothing and bandages. Most patients feel no sensations during the procedure.

When is Magnetic Therapy Prescribed?
Magnetic therapy is effective for treating various conditions, including:

1. Bronchopulmonary System: Respiratory issues.
2. Musculoskeletal System: Bruises, hematomas, bone fractures, and cracks.

3. Central Nervous System: Neurological issues.

4. Digestive Organs: Digestive problems.

5. Cardiovascular System: Heart and blood vessel conditions.

6. Skin: Dermatitis, neurodermatitis.

7. Peripheral Vessels: Issues with blood vessels.

8. Delayed Speech Development: Especially with the "Headband" attachment.

Pediatric Physiotherapy: The "Headband" Attachment

The "Headband" is used for transcranial magnetic therapy, which involves a traveling pulsed magnetic field. It has several therapeutic effects:

1. Deep Brain Impact: Affects deep brain structures.

2. Nerve Conduction: Improves nerve impulse transmission.

3. Vasodilation: Widens blood vessels.

4. Microcirculation: Enhances blood flow in the hypothalamic-pituitary region.

5. Liquor Dynamics: Improves cerebrospinal fluid movement.

Indications for "Headband" Use in Pediatrics:

1. Cerebrovascular Issues: Blood flow problems in the brain.

2. Post-Traumatic Injuries: After brain injuries (e.g., asthenoneurotic syndrome, vascular dystonia).

3. Headaches: Chronic or acute headaches.

4. Nerve Disorders: Neuralgia and neuropathy (e.g., trigeminal, facial nerves).

5. Optic Nerve Atrophy: Partial vision loss.

6. Amblyopia: Lazy eye condition.

7. Visual Analyzer Dysfunction: Vision problems.

8. Hydrocephalic Syndrome: Increased intracranial pressure.

9. Obesity: Especially hypothalamic obesity.

10. ENT Pathology: Frequent ear, nose, and throat issues and allergic rhinitis.

11. Gastrointestinal Disorders: IBS, reflux esophagitis.

12. Skin Conditions: Neurodermatitis, atopic dermatitis.

13. Puberty Issues: Hypothalamic syndrome during puberty.

Procedure and Safety

The pediatric magnetic therapy procedure is safe and effective, complementing other physiotherapeutic treatments. Each session lasts 15-20 minutes, and a full treatment course can include up to 20 sessions, depending on the child's condition and age.

Magnetic therapy is an effective and reliable method in pediatric physiotherapy, helping to treat a variety of conditions safely.

Magnetic Therapy for Osteochondrosis of the Spine

Chronic spine diseases are a major concern in modern medicine. One of these conditions, osteochondrosis, involves degenerative changes in the spine. Treating this condition requires a comprehensive approach to relieve symptoms, prevent flare-ups, and improve the patient's overall quality of life. Magnetic therapy offers an alternative conservative treatment for osteochondrosis.

What is Osteochondrosis?

Osteochondrosis involves the breakdown and degeneration of spinal discs and joints. It's worth noting that many people show signs of osteochondrosis on imaging tests without experiencing back pain. Conversely, back pain symptoms are not always due to osteochondrosis.

How Magnetic Therapy Works

The body's systems respond differently to magnetic fields. Here's the order of sensitivity:

1. Nervous System
2. Endocrine System
3. Sensory Organs
4. Cardiovascular System
5. Digestive System
6. Urinary System
7. Respiratory System
8. Musculoskeletal System

Magnetic therapy is unique because magnetic fields are naturally part of the human body.

Benefits of Magnetic Therapy for the Spine

Magnetic therapy can provide several benefits for spinal health:

- Improves Capillary Blood Flow: Enhances circulation in small blood vessels.

- Normalizes Vascular Permeability: Stabilizes blood vessel walls.

- Restores Cell Polarity: Rebalances cells and their contents.

- Activates Enzyme Systems: Boosts the body's natural enzyme functions.

When applied to the musculoskeletal system, magnetic fields increase the concentration of iron ions in bone tissue. Copper levels also rise, which is crucial for cellular reactions, activating the body's adaptive responses. Additionally, the increased activity of magnesium improves muscle tone.

Indications for Magnetic Therapy

Magnetic therapy should be used as part of a comprehensive treatment plan and prescribed by a doctor after evaluating the patient's condition. Here are common reasons for using magnetic therapy:

- Muscle Stiffness: Reduces tightness and improves flexibility.

- Acute Inflammation: Eases inflammation in the spine.

- Chronic Pain: Helps when acute pain becomes chronic.

- Dizziness and Visual Disturbances: Alleviates symptoms like dizziness, spots, and tinnitus.

- Spinal Pain: Addresses pain in any part of the spine.

- Sensory and Motor Impairments: Improves sensation and movement.

- Spinal "Crunching": Reduces unusual sounds or feelings when turning.

In summary, magnetic therapy is a valuable tool for managing osteochondrosis and other spine-related conditions, providing multiple therapeutic benefits while being a part of a broader treatment strategy.

Magnetic Therapy for Osteochondrosis

Magnetic therapy has shown promising results in treating osteochondrosis, particularly during periods of acute inflammation with noticeable symptoms. Studies reveal its effectiveness, especially when other treatments fail to provide relief.

Benefits of Magnetic Therapy

1. Pain Relief: It effectively reduces acute pain and discomfort associated with osteochondrosis.

2. Tissue Health: Magnetic therapy promotes healing and improves tissue health in the musculoskeletal system, potentially preventing future flare-ups.

3. Improved Well-being: Patients report overall improvement, not just in pain, but also in other neurological symptoms like dizziness, headaches, and tinnitus.

Combination Therapy

Combining magnetic therapy with laser therapy has gained popularity recently. This approach enhances the therapeutic effects and can provide more significant relief. The indications and contraindications remain the same, but the combined therapy often yields better results.

Contraindications and Side Effects

While magnetic therapy offers benefits, it's essential to use it under medical supervision due to its potential side effects. Contraindications include bleeding disorders, cancer, severe vascular damage, and certain medical implants. Side effects like local allergic reactions or mild discomfort may occur, but they are rare and usually temporary.

Procedure

Magnetic therapy is non-invasive and painless. The patient lies comfortably on a treatment table while the physiotherapist places flexible magnetic applicators on the skin, secured with bandages. The session typically lasts 15-20 minutes, with the first session shorter as a precaution against adverse reactions. The physiotherapist monitors the progress closely to ensure safety and effectiveness.

In summary, magnetic therapy offers a promising approach to managing osteochondrosis, providing relief from pain and promoting tissue healing without invasive procedures.

Number of Procedures in Magnetic Therapy

The number of sessions and the intensity of magnetic therapy vary based on the patient's condition and the doctor's assessment.

Typically, a full course of magnetic therapy consists of 20 sessions, but this can vary.

For some patients, especially those without contraindications, a shorter course of 5-7 sessions may be sufficient. When combined with other treatments, such as medications or physical therapy, fewer sessions, usually 1-3, may be recommended.

During the procedure, most patients don't experience any discomfort. However, depending on the equipment used, they may feel a slight vibration or warmth. In some cases, stronger settings may cause muscle contractions or tingling sensations, which are usually tolerable.

Magnetic therapy is a versatile and painless treatment for osteochondrosis and spinal column issues. It often produces positive results, even when other treatments have failed. It's essential to discuss all available options with the patient to determine the best approach for both treatment and prevention of the disease.

Low-Frequency Magnetic Therapy Explained

Low-frequency magnetic therapy is a commonly used treatment where low-frequency magnetic fields are employed for therapeutic, preventive, and rehabilitative purposes. This type of therapy affects the nervous, cardiovascular, and endocrine systems of the body in beneficial ways.

Low-frequency magnetic fields can increase nerve impulse transmission speed, reduce nerve swelling, normalize blood clotting, stimulate metabolism, and enhance regeneration processes. Some studies even suggest it may have an antitumor effect in certain cancers.

This therapy stimulates tissue regeneration by boosting blood flow and nutrient delivery, particularly benefiting nervous tissue. It can also improve blood flow and lower blood pressure by relaxing blood vessel spasms.

Indications for Use

Low-frequency magnetic therapy is recommended for various conditions, including:

- Cardiovascular issues like hypertension and coronary heart disease
- Hormonal imbalances
- Chronic digestive disorders such as ulcers
- Musculoskeletal problems like osteochondrosis and arthritis

It can enhance overall well-being, increase resistance to radiation, and improve the body's ability to adapt.

Contraindications

However, it's essential to note some contraindications, including:

- Acute heart problems
- Bleeding disorders
- Pregnancy
- Cancerous growths
- High body temperature

How the Procedure Works

During the therapy, the affected area and surrounding tissues are heated slightly, promoting increased blood flow, reduced inflammation, improved immunity, and enhanced healing mechanisms.

There are different methods of applying magnetic therapy, including contact, labile, and remote control. Sometimes, it's administered vaginally or rectally for specific conditions.

Procedure Guidelines

To ensure effectiveness and safety, follow these guidelines:

- Avoid alcohol before sessions.

- Don't undergo therapy on an empty or full stomach.

- Maintain a regular schedule for sessions.

- Rest for 30-60 minutes after each session.

- Avoid therapy during illness, low blood pressure, or after taking certain medications.

By adhering to these rules, low-frequency magnetic therapy can be a valuable addition to treatment plans for various conditions, offering relief and promoting healing.

Using Magnets to Kill Cancer

Understanding Cancer

Cancer remains a significant health challenge worldwide, causing millions of deaths annually. While science progresses, finding effective treatments for cancer is complex due to its unknown nature. We understand cancer is caused by genetic mutations, but identifying the precise triggers remains elusive.

Current Treatments and Challenges

Standard cancer treatments involve surgery, radiation therapy, and chemotherapy. While effective, they can lead to prolonged recovery and adverse side effects, impacting patients physically and emotionally.

The Promise of Magnetic Therapy

Alternative treatments aim to target cancer cells while minimizing harm to healthy tissue and the immune system. Magnetic therapy emerges as a potential approach.

Magnetic Therapy and Cancer Cells

Studies explore how magnets could combat cancer. Magnetic therapy offers minimal invasiveness, reducing the need for surgery and minimizing harm to healthy tissues.

Experimental Studies

In one study, mice with breast cancer cells were exposed to magnetic fields, leading to suppressed tumor growth and cancer cell death through apoptosis, a natural cell death process.

Magnetic Hyperthermia

Another promising method involves magnetic nanoparticles combined with hyperthermia therapy. Hyperthermia utilizes high temperatures to destroy cancer cells, often combined with radiation or chemotherapy.

Research Findings

Studies show magnetic nanoparticles, when activated by alternating magnetic fields, can generate heat, effectively killing cancer cells. The effectiveness depends on factors like nanoparticle size and composition.

Future Directions

Further research is needed to understand the optimal application of magnetic therapy for cancer treatment. Investigating factors like exposure intensity and duration can enhance treatment outcomes.

In conclusion, while magnetic therapy shows promise, more research is essential to unlock its full potential in cancer treatment. By delving deeper into its mechanisms and applications, we move closer to more effective cancer therapies.

Magnetic Therapy for Alzheimer's Disease

Understanding Obsessive-Compulsive Disorder (OCD)

Obsessive-compulsive disorder (OCD) is a mental health condition characterized by obsessive thoughts and repetitive behaviors. While not as severe as some mental illnesses, OCD can significantly impact a person's daily life, self-esteem, and social interactions.

Research on Magnetic Nanoparticles

Scientists investigated the use of magnetic nanoparticles to activate cellular receptors in the brain associated with pain and heat sensation. In an experiment with rodents, low-frequency magnetic fields were applied to the brain after delivering magnetic nanoparticles to specific areas. This non-invasive method showed promise in stimulating neurons without side effects.

Potential Applications in Alzheimer's Disease

While the focus was on OCD, this technology's success opens doors for broader applications, including Alzheimer's disease. By understanding how magnetic particles affect brain function, researchers aim to develop targeted therapies for various neurological conditions.

Understanding Magnetotherapy

Magnetotherapy is a form of physiotherapy that uses magnetic fields to treat various diseases. Unlike traditional therapies, magnetotherapy is non-invasive and offers adjustable intensity levels. It has gained popularity due to its effectiveness and convenience.

How Magnetotherapy Works

During magnetotherapy, pulsed magnetic fields are directed at the affected area, promoting blood vessel dilation and reducing inflammation and pain. It can also improve tissue oxygenation and accelerate healing. This makes it a promising treatment option for genitourinary system diseases.

Treatment Process

Magnetotherapy devices emit magnetic fields through inductors placed on the affected area. Treatment sessions typically last 20-30 minutes, with 10-14 sessions recommended for a full course. Sessions can be conducted daily or every other day, with the option for repeat courses if needed.

Research and Future Directions

Ongoing research aims to deepen our understanding of magnetotherapy's mechanisms and its potential applications. While some skepticism remains due to its relatively recent emergence, continued studies seek to provide more evidence of its effectiveness in treating various conditions, including Alzheimer's disease.

Research has shown that magnetic therapy can effectively reduce muscle tension around the spine and treat neurovascular issues. By restoring blood circulation and slowing down the degeneration of intervertebral discs, magnetic therapy offers relief from pain. Patients often report an improvement in their overall well-being after undergoing a series of magnetic therapy sessions.

During the procedure, magnetic fields target the spine, enhancing microcirculation and providing cells with essential nutrients. With minimal contraindications and high effectiveness, magnetic therapy has become a valuable treatment option for various musculoskeletal problems. It is commonly used alongside other conservative treatments but can also be utilized independently.

After the therapy session, patients experience a decrease in pain as the tissues surrounding the inflamed areas of the spine become less swollen, restoring mobility to the vertebrae. Additionally, low-frequency magnetic field exposure helps dilate blood vessels, reduce blood viscosity, and enhance oxygen metabolism in tissues, further contributing to pain relief and overall improvement in musculoskeletal health.

In conclusion, magnetic therapy shows promise as a non-invasive treatment option for Alzheimer's disease and other neurological conditions. Further research and advancements in this field hold the potential to improve the lives of individuals affected by these debilitating illnesses.

Using Magnetic Therapy for Neurological Diseases

The Research Institute of Emergency Medicine, named after I.I. Janelidze, is actively employing rhythmic transcranial magnetic stimulation (rTMS) in the treatment of patients with neurological disorders. This method has emerged as one of the most effective techniques in neurology.

Rhythmic TMS, a painless method of magnetic brain stimulation, has demonstrated safety and efficacy since its introduction in the late 1990s. Diana Vladimirovna Tokareva, a physiotherapist at the Institute's medical rehabilitation department, highlights its versatility for various patient conditions, provided there are no contraindications.

Indications for using this method include:

- Rehabilitating motor disorders post-stroke.
- Treating speech disorders like aphasia.
- Addressing neglect syndrome.
- Managing dysphagia (swallowing difficulties).
- Alleviating migraine and complex regional pain syndrome.
- Managing neuropathic pain and tinnitus.
- Addressing psychiatric diseases.

Transpinal magnetic stimulation, a form of rhythmic magnetic stimulation, targets spinal cord structures. It can also affect peripheral nerve structures, such as nerves affected by neuropathies or injuries.

However, certain precautions must be observed. Absolute contraindications include the presence of electronic implanted devices, such as pacemakers or pumps, in the patient's body. Relative contraindications involve conditions like epilepsy or pregnancy. After traumatic brain injury or hemorrhagic stroke, caution is advised, and electroencephalography may be necessary before proceeding with treatment.

The effects of rhythmic transpinal magnetic stimulation can be immediate or delayed. Determining the suitability of rTMS and the duration of therapy is done during in-person consultations with medical rehabilitation specialists.

Treating Spinal Hernia with Magnetic Therapy

A spinal hernia, a serious condition of the musculoskeletal system, can cause significant discomfort and restrict movement. It typically occurs in the lower back but can affect other parts of the spine too.

A hernia forms when the fibrous ring around an intervertebral disc ruptures, causing the disc's core to protrude and put pressure on nerves and tissues. This often leads to intense back pain, which can worsen with activity or even at rest.

Magnetic therapy, a modern and effective treatment, uses a low-frequency magnetic field to improve the patient's well-being and speed up their recovery.

Indications and Contraindications for Magnetic Therapy

Magnetic therapy is beneficial for patients with various musculoskeletal conditions and is often used to prevent complications. It's recommended for conditions such as limited limb mobility, tissue swelling around the hernia, muscle spasms, urinary system issues, inflammation, poor blood flow to the legs, loss of sensation, and pain of any intensity.

However, while magnetic therapy is effective, there are some limitations to consider. It's not suitable for individuals with malignant cancers, pregnancy, implanted pacemakers or metal implants, recent heart attacks, severe heart conditions, acute infections, bleeding disorders, autoimmune diseases, purulent infections, high fevers, adrenal gland issues, severe mental illnesses, high blood pressure, advanced tuberculosis, or blood clotting issues.

How Magnetic Therapy Works for Spinal Hernia

Magnetic therapy impacts the body's lymphatic and circulatory systems, enhancing microcirculation in tissue capillaries. This process boosts cell nutrition, oxygen supply, and toxin removal, promoting tissue renewal and regeneration. For spinal hernia, magnetic therapy can reduce tissue swelling and inflammation, alleviate pain, relax back muscles, relieve nerve root compression, restore mobility, and improve blood flow to the affected area. It also enhances the absorption of medications injected into the tissue.

Types of Magnetic Therapy Devices

Magnetic therapy can be administered through various devices:

1. Professional devices: They treat the entire body.

2. Micromagnets: Small buttons attached to the body's bioactive points.

3. Special tape recorders: Rubberized plates with built-in magnets, worn with a comfortable belt or corset.

Micromagnets provide targeted therapy without risking cell damage, offering effective pain relief and improved tissue nutrition.

Combining Therapies

Treating spinal hernia often requires a combination of therapies, including magnetic therapy, physiotherapy, targeted exercises, and medication. By integrating these approaches, patients can experience significant relief and promote healing.

Improving Vision with Magnetic Therapy

Magnetic therapy involves using a constant or alternating magnetic field to prevent and treat various conditions. During a session, the body's charged particles interact with the magnetic field, providing anti-inflammatory and pain-relieving effects. The most effective treatment involves an alternating magnetic field, which requires less tension and shorter exposure time. One of the significant advantages of magnetic therapy is that it doesn't require direct contact with the radiation source, making the procedure painless. Patients might only hear quiet sound signals indicating the generation of magnetic pulses.

Conditions Treated with Magnetic Therapy for Vision

Magnetic therapy can help treat several eye conditions, including:

- Glaucoma (in the early stages)
- Myopia, hyperopia, astigmatism, and presbyopia
- Retinal dystrophy
- Corneal erosion
- Inflammatory eye diseases (conjunctivitis, blepharitis, keratitis, uveitis)
- Eye swelling
- Postoperative complications
- Optic nerve partial atrophy
- Various forms of keratitis
- Spasms of accommodation
- Eye hemorrhages
- Endocrine eye disorders
- Iridocyclitis and episcleritis

- Retinal ischemia

Under magnetic therapy, blood vessels dilate, blood circulation improves, cell regeneration accelerates, muscles relax, and anti-inflammatory effects occur.

Therapeutic Effects of Magnetic Therapy
Magnetic therapy provides several therapeutic benefits:

- Relieving eye strain, particularly beneficial for those who spend long hours in front of screens or driving, by relaxing muscles and reducing fatigue
- Aiding in eye injury recovery by reducing swelling and promoting wound healing, including corneal damage
- Lowering intraocular pressure

- Resolving exudate, infiltrates, and intraocular hemorrhages, as well as reducing inflammation and swelling
- Accelerating metabolic processes and improving blood circulation, especially in the retina
- Relaxing eye muscles and improving blood and lymph microcirculation around the eyes

After a course of magnetic therapy, patients often experience improved vision and better eye health. However, it's essential to consider contraindications before undergoing treatment.

Contraindications for Magnetic Therapy

Despite its benefits, magnetic therapy may not be suitable for individuals with certain conditions, including:

- Cardiovascular diseases

- Low blood pressure

- Tuberculosis or hyperthyroidism

- Thrombosis

- Mental disorders

- Cancer

- Hemorrhages

- Acute infections

If any of these conditions are present, magnetic therapy should be avoided unless a healthcare professional advises otherwise. It's crucial to consult with a doctor before undergoing magnetic therapy to ensure its safety and effectiveness for individual cases.

Performing Magnetic Therapy for Vision Treatment

In modern medicine, there are numerous devices that emit low-frequency magnetic pulses, making magnetic therapy a common method for treating eye conditions. The choice of device depends on factors such as the patient's age and the type of disorder. A typical course of treatment involves 10-15 sessions, each lasting 7-10 minutes. There's no need to disrupt one's daily routine or take sick leave for these sessions, as they can be easily integrated into regular activities. During the session, the patient sits in front of the device while the ophthalmologist adjusts the treatment mode. The magnetic field inductor is placed directly in front of the affected eye, and the procedure can be performed through a gauze bandage.

Effectiveness of Magnetophoresis

A particularly effective method is magnetophoresis, where specific eye medications are administered under the influence of a magnetic field. For example, Taufon, an eye drop containing taurine, is used for treating cataracts, corneal diseases, glaucoma, and eye injuries. Taurine promotes eye tissue regeneration, reduces intraocular pressure, strengthens blood vessels, and prevents retinal issues. When combined with magnetic therapy, the effectiveness of Taufon is enhanced as the magnetic waves help push the drug molecules into the eye tissue.

Magnetic Therapy for Children's Vision

Magnetic therapy is also commonly used to treat various eye disorders in children, including amblyopia, strabismus, and myopia. Myopia, or nearsightedness, is particularly prevalent in childhood, and timely treatment can yield positive results. Magnetic therapy reduces eye fatigue, improves vision clarity and accommodation, and can halt the progression of myopia. Devices like the AMO-ATOS magnetic pulse device, often used in ophthalmology clinics, are effective for treating children's vision issues. These devices, along with special attachments like "Amblio," achieve a significant therapeutic effect by reducing spasm, inflammation, and swelling in the eyes, improving blood circulation, and normalizing intraocular fluid outflow.

Magnetic therapy for children is often designed to be enjoyable, resembling a game, and is completely painless and safe when there are no contraindications. Treatment plans are tailored to each child's specific eye condition and age, ensuring optimal results.

Home Magnetotherapy for Vision

Apart from devices found in clinics, there are portable magnetic devices available for home use. These devices, manufactured by Russian companies and certified for use, can provide magnetic therapy conveniently at home. However, it's crucial not to decide on their use independently. Only after consulting with an ophthalmologist can magnetic therapy for vision be approved for home treatment.

Home hardware treatment is often suggested for individuals with weakened immune systems and elderly patients. Once the specialist approves this therapy, it's important to carefully read the instructions for use to achieve the best results. A typical course usually involves 10-15 sessions, and no more than three such courses should be conducted within a year. It's advisable to perform the procedure before bedtime, while resting. The duration of the sessions should be determined independently, starting with a short period but not exceeding the time specified in the instructions.

When purchasing portable devices for home treatment, it's recommended to buy them from specialized stores, either retail or online, that sell medical equipment. Avoid trusting excessively low prices and purchasing from unfamiliar websites.

Chapter 6

Indications and Contraindications of

Magnetic Therapy

Indications for Magnetic Therapy:

Physiotherapeutic procedures using magnetic waves find applications across various medical fields. Some primary indications include:

1. **Nervous System Disorders:** This includes conditions like chronic circulatory disorders, traumatic brain injuries, post-

stroke conditions, impaired motor activity, and nerve inflammations.

2. Musculoskeletal System Disorders: Magnetic therapy is beneficial for soft tissue bruises, degenerative joint changes, bone fractures, muscle atrophy, and arthritis.

3. Heart and Blood Vessel Pathologies: It can help with high blood pressure, heart muscle ischemia, heart failure, and atherosclerotic changes in blood vessels.

4. Digestive System Diseases: Conditions like ulceration or erosion of the digestive tract mucous membrane, bile excretion issues, gastritis, and chronic inflammation of the pancreas or liver.

5.   Respiratory   System   Pathologies:
Magnetic therapy is effective for pneumonia, bronchial asthma, and chronic inflammation of the paranasal sinuses.

6. Genitourinary System Disorders: It can assist in treating chronic prostatitis, erectile dysfunction, kidney stones, and inflammation of female genital organs.

Orthopedic and urological practices frequently utilize magnetic therapy due to its high demand.

Contraindications:
However, magnetic therapy isn't suitable for all patients, and there are certain contraindications to consider:

1. Severe Heart and Blood Vessel Pathologies: Conditions such as severe heart diseases and blood vessel disorders may pose risks with magnetic therapy.

2. Malignant Neoplasms: Patients with malignant tumors are typically not suitable candidates for magnetic therapy.

3. Immunopathological Disorders: Those with disorders affecting the immune system may have adverse reactions to magnetic therapy.

4. Severe Body Exhaustion: Individuals experiencing severe physical exhaustion due to illness may not benefit from magnetic therapy.

5. Other Conditions: Atherosclerosis of cerebral arteries, acute infections, unexplained fever, abnormal blood coagulation, and hematological disorders are also contraindications.

It's essential for the doctor to carefully review the patient's medical history and rule out any contraindications before proceeding with magnetic therapy. Additionally, specific devices may have their own limitations, so reading the instructions beforehand is crucial.

www.ingramcontent.com/pod-product-compliance
Lightning Source LLC
Chambersburg PA
CBHW061245250726
48653CB00002B/518